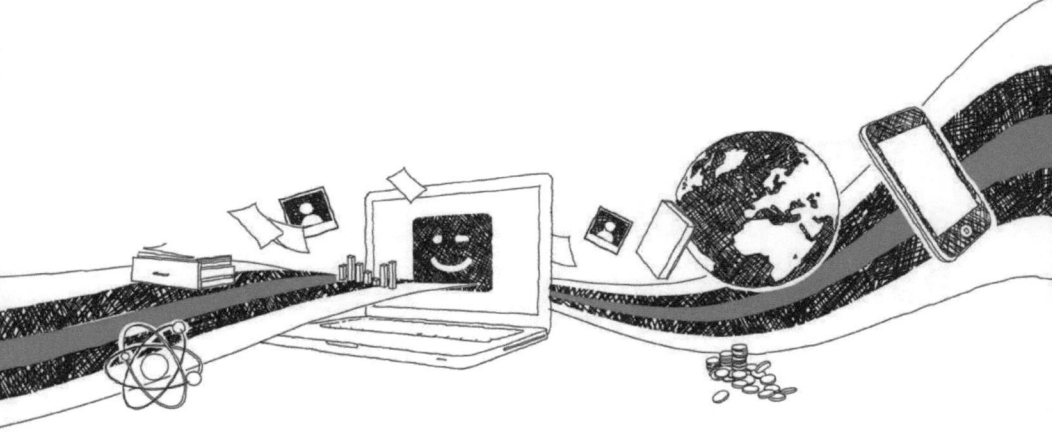
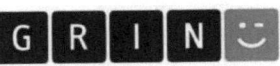

Using a Winogradsky Column to enrich microbes as they are by simulating various conditions and to predict Microcosm Biofilm Patterns using time lapse tracing and regression analysis

T.S. Amar Anand Rao

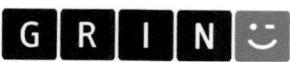

Bibliographic information published by the German National Library:

The German National Library lists this publication in the National Bibliography; detailed bibliographic data are available on the Internet at http://dnb.dnb.de.

ISBN: 9783656090670
This book is also available as an ebook.

© GRIN Publishing GmbH
Trappentreustraße 1
80339 München

Print and binding: Books on Demand GmbH, Norderstedt, Germany
Printed on acid-free paper from responsible sources.

The present work has been carefully prepared. Nevertheless, authors and publishers do not incur liability for the correctness of information, notes, links and advice as well as any printing errors.

GRIN web shop: https://www.grin.com/document/184263

Using a Winogradsky Column to Enrich microbes as they are by Simulating various conditions and to Predict Microcosm Biofilm Patterns using time lapse tracing and regression analysis

T.S. Amar Anand Rao

Molecular Biophysics Unit, Indian Institute of Science

Bangalore – 560012, Karnataka, India.

Abstract

Of all the microbes known most are uncultured because of their fastidious nature . Most part of microbial interactions are still unexplored. Herein we use an age old tool, Winogradsky column to enrich, simulate the microbes as they are and predict microcosm biofilm patterns. We have worked on many simulation parameters to better the Winogradsky column in every way. We describe methods to bring the interactions of the microbes in biofilms at a mathematical level. We also have explored the various practical applications possible out of winogradsky column like using it as a universal enrichment medium for all microbes to grow as they are and also to isolate and evolve purpose based microbes for degradation studies, harnessing the redox potential of microbial succession.

Keywords

Winogradsky Column/ Microcosm/   Biofilm/ microbial succession/ simulation/   degradation/ nutrient cycle/ regression

Introduction

The Winogradsky column is a glass or clear plastic column, filled with enriched soil or sedi- ment. When developed, it has an anaerobic lower zone and aerobic upper zone that allow growth of microorganisms under conditions similar to those found in sediments and water rich in nutrients (Sylvia et al., 1998).

Often teachers simply convey the message that different microorganisms exist in different strata of the column and that some live in the aerobic and some in anaerobic zones. However, this is really where the discovery begins rather than ends! Explaining the complexity that lies within the depths of the ecosystem allows deeper insights into the microbial world (Rogan et al., 2005).

Construction and development of Winogradsky column incorporates several variables. With just a few changes, different columns can be created to compare growth rates, microbial populations, and ecological diversity (Rogan et al., 2005)

In each experiment, set up one winogradsky column to serve as a control. This column will be the standard and each of the other columns should vary in only one aspect, such as concentration of a given pesticide from the control column. The results in the column may be obtained by observing the colour changes within the columns. Each change represents the activity of a different group of microorganisms. The sequence of events in the winogradsky column may take as little as six weeks to two months under warm conditions. Under cooler conditions, the reactions will occur more slowly. The succession observed by Kobyashy and Okuda (Hattori 1973) in a column containing soil and water from a rice paddy required two and a half months and occured in this order: 1)green algae (green appeared in about one week); 2) sulphate reducing bacteria (black) were evident at four weeks; 3) photosynthetic purple bacteria (red) appeared five to six weeks later; and, 4) the purple non sulphur bacteria (green) were seen within the next few weeks. The winogradsky column can be a useful tool to demonstrate succession and microbial interdependence with relative ease and simplicity. Also we can follow the chemical reactions and recycling of material within the column to gain an understanding of how they occur in nature (Pigage et al., 1985)

The Winogradsky column was developed and named after Sergei Winogradsky (1856-1953), a Russian microbiologist. He studied the complex interactions between environmental conditions and microbial activities using soil enrichment to isolate pure bacterial cultures (Madigan et al., 2000)

Over one hundred years ago, Sergei Winogradsky studied the microbial organisms inhabiting sulphide-rich black mud ecosystems and pioneered our understanding of chemolithotrophy through his experiments with sulphate and nitrate reducing organisms. Although many of the microbes from black mud environments (which are often used to inoculate so-called "Winogradsky columns") have been studied for decades, the vast majority of the microorganisms present in natural black mud ecosystems remain unknown to microbiologists. While the physiology and biochemistry of microorganisms are best studied in pure cultures, this may prove very tedious in the case of black mud microbes, because the complex community has co-evolved for millions of years. Syntrophy -- the requirement of a microbe to associate with another microbial species for metabolites -- is probably critical to the survival of most of the species within this complex environment (Tanner et al., 2000)

An excellent but perhaps overlooked tool for the study of microbial activity in the soil, nutrient cycling, microbial succession and ecology is the Winogradsky column (Pigage et al., 1985)

What we have done is a time lapse trace of biofilm patterns in the Winogradsky column, taking equivalent weights of each biofilm patterns by cutting the traces of biofilms and weighing them individually and then using regression equations to estimate the biomass with time. Thus over a period of time we were able to give a regression coefficient to each of the coloured pattern in the column and hence give a simulation and prediction tool.

Materials and Methods

Sample Collection

Pond soil and water were collected from the water soil interphase of ponds at Government Botanical Gardens, Ooty. This place was selected because these gardens have been undisturbed natural biosphere (Figure 2).

Procedure of making a Winogradsky column (Anderson et al 1999) the soil sample was cleaned of debris, stones, pebbles, grass clippings, leaves and moving insects. This is used as the control column and standard reference (Figure 3).

1. Fill one fourth of a 250ml glass measuring cylinder with the soil.
2. Mix the soil with 2g of cellulose, 2g of calcium carbonate, and 2g of calcium sulphate.
3. Cover upto three fourth of the column with soil slurry.
4. Let the soil set for five minutes to release trapped air bubbles.
5. Add water leaving a 2cm gap at top.
6. Incubate the column where it will receive daylight or artificial light.

7. Observe the column over the next several weeks for development of layers, smell, colours, and zones.

Simulation of varied environmental factors

By building variations of Winogradsky column one factor at a time- other conditions were kept unchanged.

Variations of nutrients

Column 1 contains carbon source only: 2 g cellulose

Column 2 contains sulphur source only: 2g $CaSO_4$

Column 3 contains carbonate source only: 2g of $CaCO_3$

Column 4 has no added nutrients at all

Variations of pH

pH values were maintained by adding buffer tablets to the water of the column.

Column 5 pH3

Column 6 pH5

Column 7 pH7

Column 8 pH9

Variations of light

In a water body, the visible light ranges from red to blue from top to bottom. To simulate the depth (with which the prevalent wavelength changes), the following colour papers were used to cover the

Column.

Column 9 black

Column 10 blue

Column 11 red

Column 12 orange

Variations of temperature

Temperatures possible in lab were used to match the environmental temperature.

Column 13 AC temperature of 25 degrees

Column 14 room temperature of around 27 degrees

Column 15 incubation temperature of 37 degrees

Column 16 outdoor temperature of 30 degrees

Variations of salinity

Winogradsky column was watered with the following values of salinity of water. It decides the osmotic pressure.

Column 17: 1% salt concentration

Column 18 : 2.5% salt concentration

Column 19 : 5% salt concentration

Column 20 : 10% salt concentration

Variations of texture

The texture of the soil decides the porosity.

Column 21 red garden soil

Column 22 sponge

Column 23 sand

Column 24 clay

Variations of hard substrates

To make degradation possible, the columns were made to contain the hard substrates as a sole source of carbon by starvation.

Column 25 coir

Column 26 dye

Column 27 naphthalein

Column 28 urea

Column 29 paraffin

Column 30 ash

Column 31 chitin

Standard control column

Column 32 contains standard winogradsky column used as control for all the other variations.

Electrochemical gradient potential

In column 33, the electrochemical gradient potential between the top and the bottom of the standard column was monitored by inserting multimeter probes (Anderson, 1999)

Pressure

Pressure increases with depth of water column. A Winogradsky set up was designed (no 34) to create pressure more than the atmospheric pressure. Using one way walves to the outlet and inlet, the pressure inside the closed column was increased by closing the outlet and suppling air through pumping using the pasteur pipette bulb attached to the inlet.

Wind and waves

A Winogradsky tank (no 35) was designed to simulate the wind through a nozzle of air pump and waves by a pedalling motor.

Isolation of Methylotrophs

Purpose: We may use 13C methanol (NMR sensitive) to grow methylotrophs and later use the lysed culture for growing our cells that express protein of interest. Idea was to substitute 13C methanol for glucose Cost effective. Sole source of carbon is methanol (column number 36).

Incubation

Incubation was done at room temperature and under artificial lighting in algal growth chambers for three months. Readings were taken at the end of each month.

Tracking biofilm pattern

The changing biofilm patterns of the Winogradsky columns were kept track by tracing the outlines of the biofilm patterns with colour markers on a rectangular piece of polythene sheet around the column (NASA quest)

Quantitative data of biofilm patterns

The biofilm patterns out on polythene sheets were cut according to the color markers and weighed on a microbalance. Thus the equivalent weights of biofilm patterns were got (NASA quest).

Biofilm pattern prediction formulae

Statistical tool chosen for prediction of past and future patterns of biofilms was done by using regression equations. This equation also fills the gaps in the scattered data and completes the regression curve.

The first step taken towards this is to establish a standard set of values observed over a period of time in a given set of simulation conditions. And then once the biomass values are got over a considerable period of time, then this data can be used to get the other parameters.

The formulae used are

a value denotes biofilm equivalent weight in grams

e value denotes time in days

$\text{mean}\,\bar{a} = \Sigma a$

n= number of readings

$\text{mean}\,\bar{e} = \Sigma e\,/\,n$

$\sigma a = \sqrt{\Sigma a^2\,/\,n - (\Sigma a)^2\,/\,n}$

$\sigma e = \sqrt{\Sigma e^2\,/\,n - (\Sigma e)^2\,/\,n}$

$r = \{ n\Sigma ae - (\Sigma a)(\Sigma e) \} / \{ \sqrt{n\Sigma a^2 - (\Sigma a)^2} \times \sqrt{n\Sigma e^2 - (\Sigma e)^2} \}$

a estimate - $\bar{a} = r \times \{\sigma a / \sigma e\} (e - \bar{e})$

e estimate - $\bar{e} = r \times \{\sigma e / \sigma a\} (a - \bar{a})$

value of r can be between -1 and +1

$r = +1$ denotes both lines coincide, it will linear in upward manner $r = -1$ denotes both lines coincide but in downward nature

$r = 0$ denotes two lines are perpendicular

Results

Effects of environmental factor variation on biofilm pattern

The biofilm patterns obtained in the columns were traced out on polythene sheets resulting in winogradsky map. Each pattern was cut and weighed periodically (Figure 17a, b).

Simulation of microbial succession

Microbial populations grew in succession in the winogradsky column kept as standard (Figure 19) . A white biofilm at the bottom at the bottom followed by black coloration of soil followed by purple and green biofilms appeared in the soil layer with green algal biofilms in the water layer (Figure 1)

Variants of the winogradsky column gave different biofilm patterns indicating that different pond microcosms can be simulated by manipulating the environmental factors. So it is worth designing a grand column where we can manipulate all factors precisely.

All results of column variations were interpreted using table. The change of patterns and the appearance and disappearance of patterns indicates the changes occuring in the microenvironments created by gradients developed according to the factors manipulated.

Nutrients

Even in limiting conditions of nutrients, green, rust, and black biofilm patterns appeared indicating their ability to survive in such conditions. Which may also mean that soil by itself has enough carbon substrates to be degraded anaerobically and start the microbial succession (Figure 4).

pH

All biofilm patterns decreased with increase in pH indicating their ability to tolerate low pH better (Figure 5)

Light

In dark regions black and a little brown biofilm patterns appeared indicating their ability of not requiring light. As the light ranges from red to blue, the biofilm patterns increases indicating the abundance of biofilm patterns at the interface regions of a water body (Figure 6).

Temperature

Regardless of varied temperatures all biofilm patterns grew well indicating their ability to adjust to a broad range of temperature (Figure 7)

Salinity

Biofilm patterns decreased with increase in salinity indicating intolerance only at high salinity(Figure 8)

Texture

Red soil and sand show good biofilm patterns indicating the respective porosities and texture of these soils to harbour most biofilm patterns (Figure 9)

Hard substrates

All hard substrate column showed slow gradual and dotted patterns of black and green biofilms in the anaerobic region, indicating evidence of the ability of biofilms to adapt and degrade any hard substrates (pollutants of human activity in water bodies) by the method of high frequency gene transfer based evolution that takes place only in biofilms (Figure 10 and 15).

Electrochemical gradient potential

The electrochemical potential probed between the top and bottom of a column plate showed increase in value from 0 to 500mV with time from 0 to 90 days indicating the ability to produce tiny amounts of electricity that may be used to light up diode bulbs (Figure 11).

Pressure

Under constant maintenance of pressure a little more than 1 atm rust and black colour biofilms patterns were dominant indicating their ability to grow in the depths of the water body (Figure 18).

Wind and waves

Wind and wave patterns of the devised Winogradsky tank showed all biofilm patterns including larval stages of invertebrates and tiny snails because of the good aeration (Figure 12 and 13)

These were sufficient evidence that if a column is designed to have all minute capacities of variation of environmental factors to bring about the specific environment of sampling water body a perfect simulation of the biofilm patterns can be achieved (Figure 14).

Isolation of Methylotrophs

A range of methlylotrophs ranging from algae to bacteria were obtained. Pink Pigmented Facultative Methylotrophs were isolated and cultured using MRS medium (Figure 16).

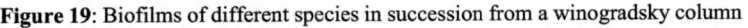
Figure 19: Biofilms of different species in succession from a winogradsky column

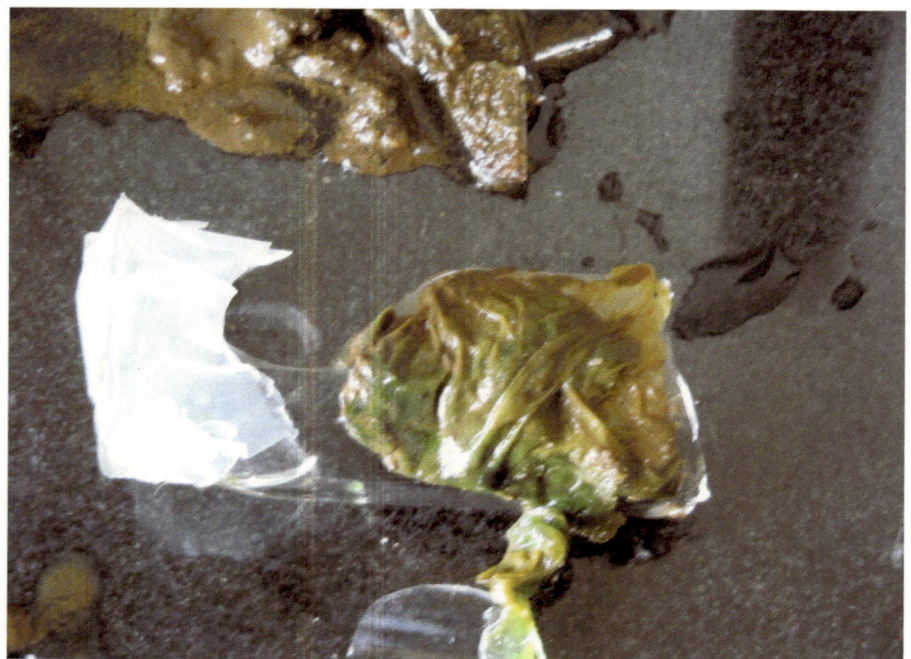

Figure 1

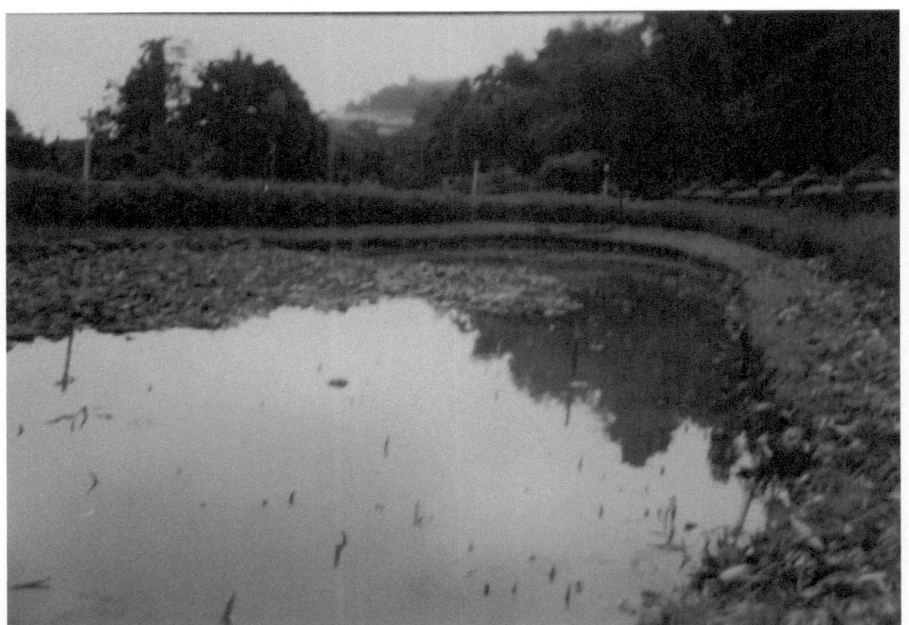

figure 2

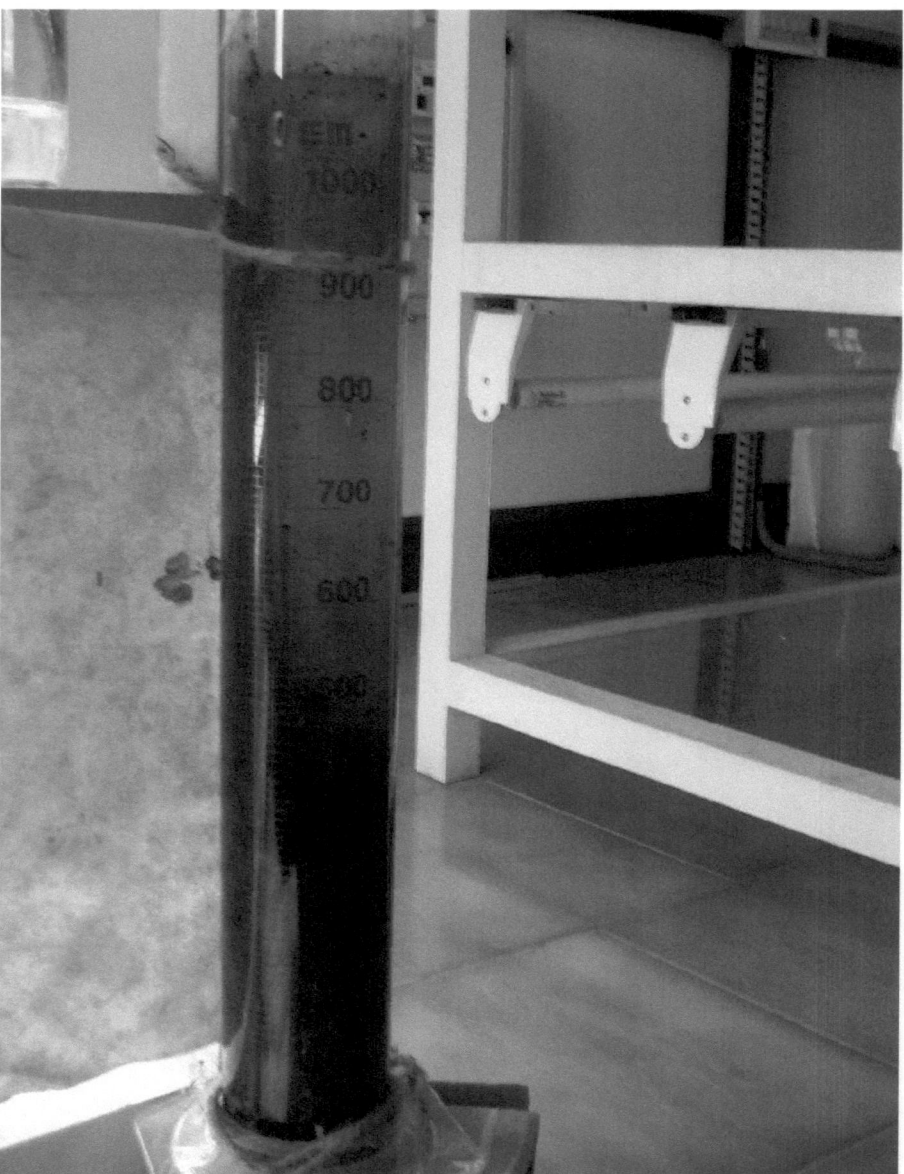

figure 3

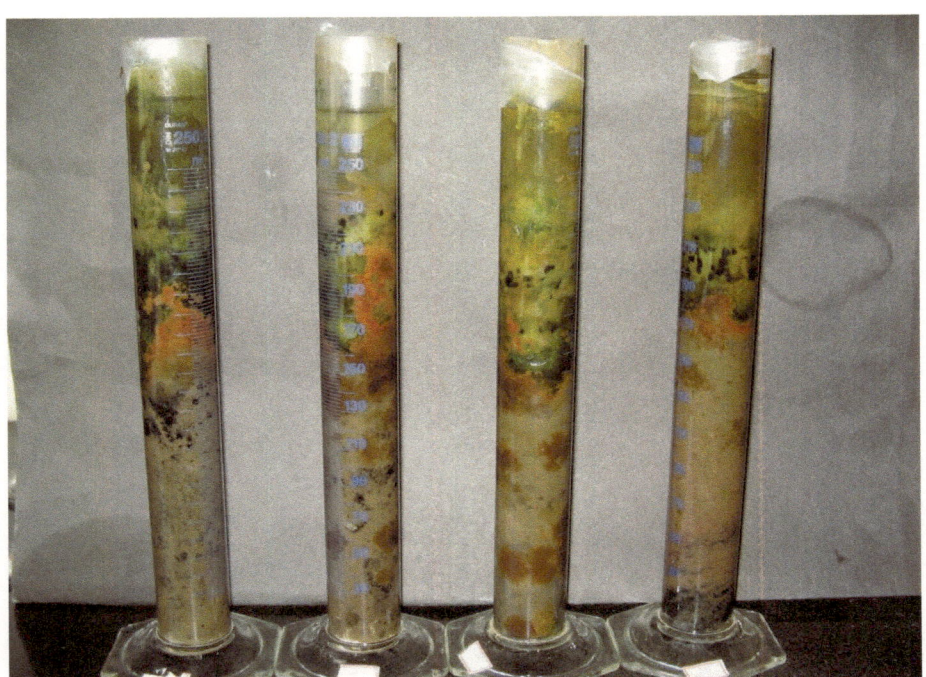

figure 4

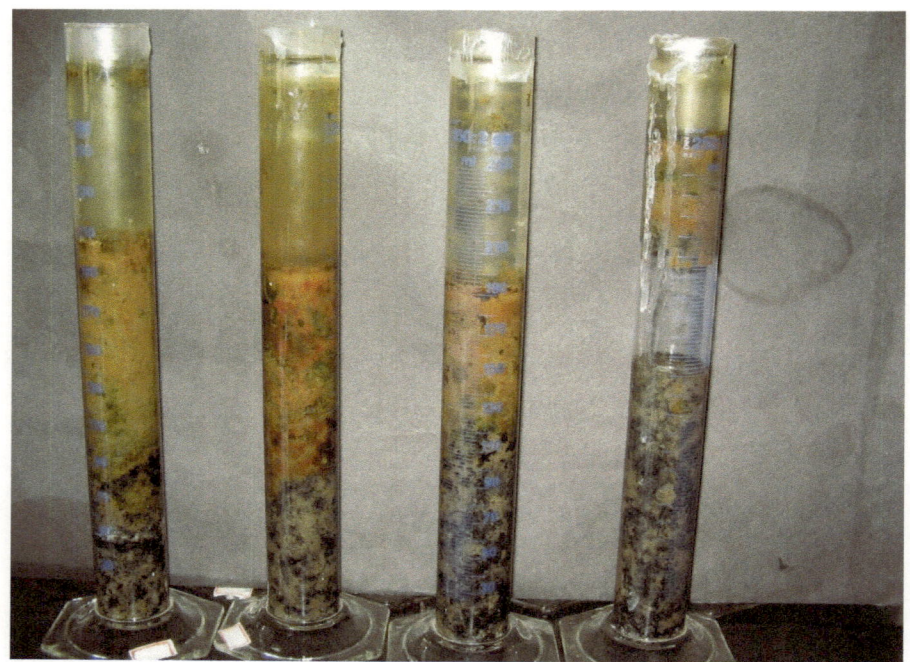

figure 5

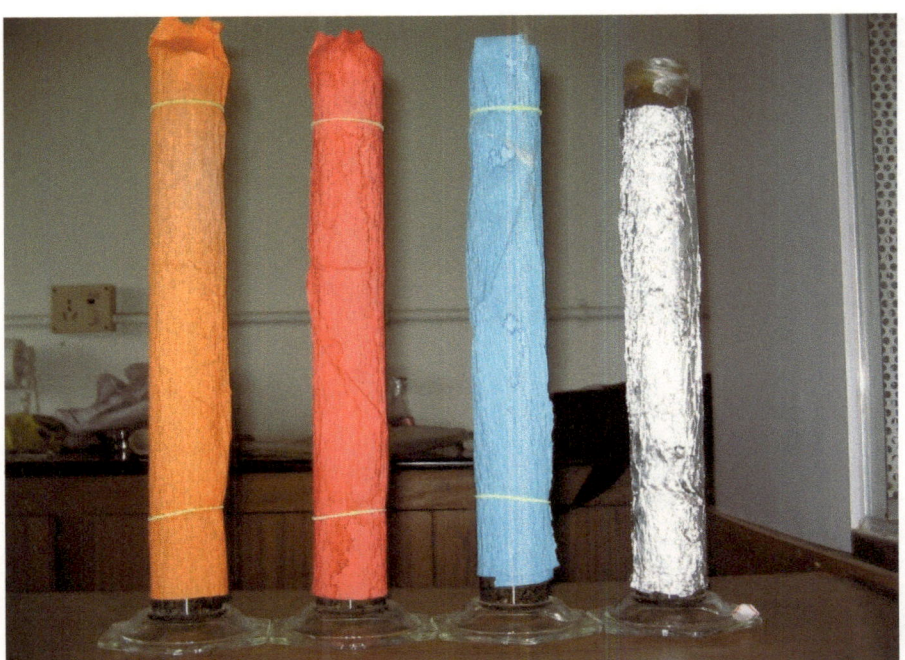

figure 6

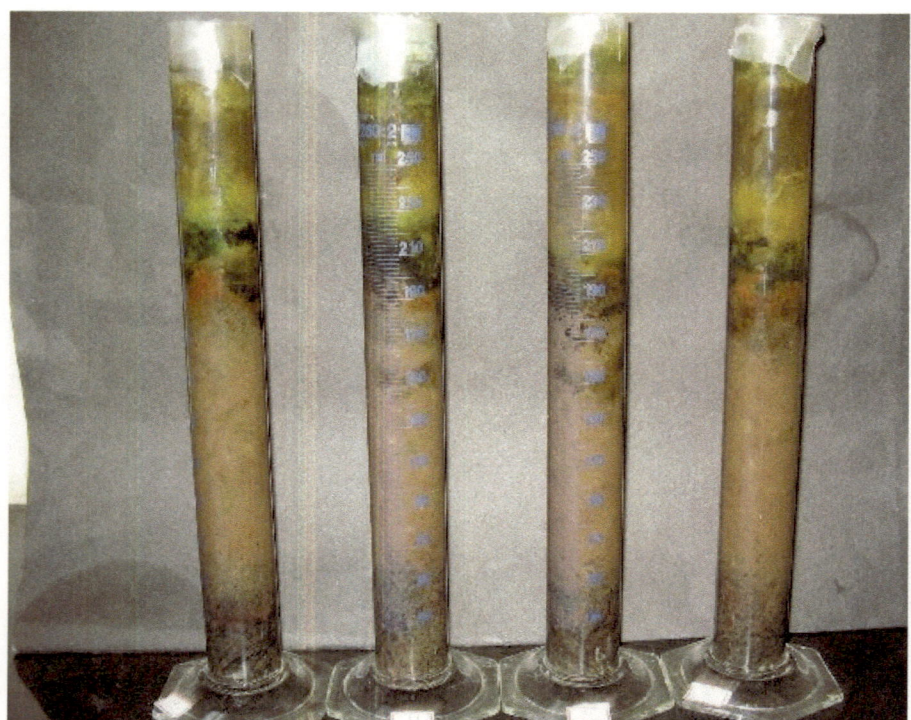

figure 7

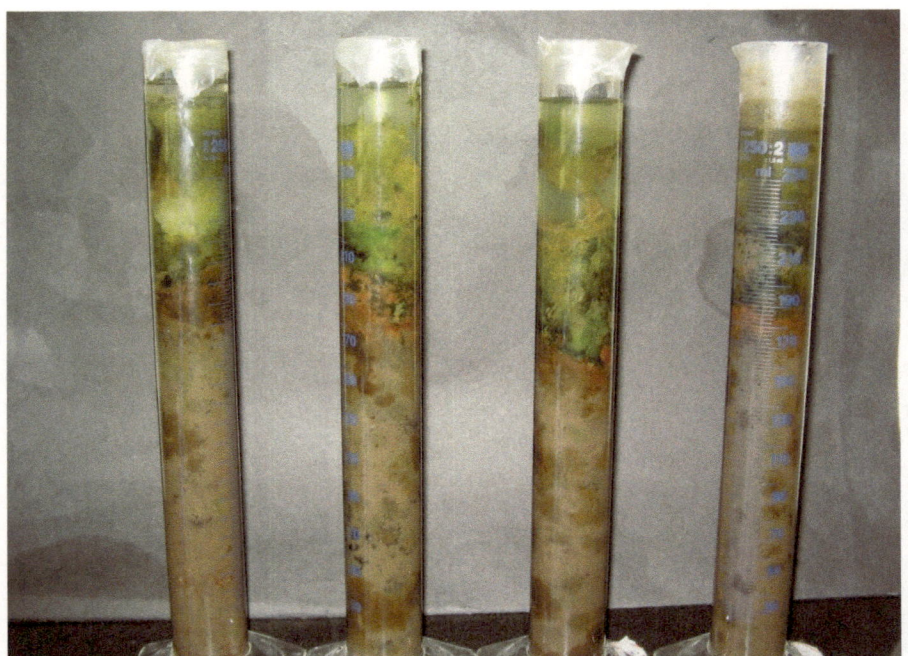
figure 8

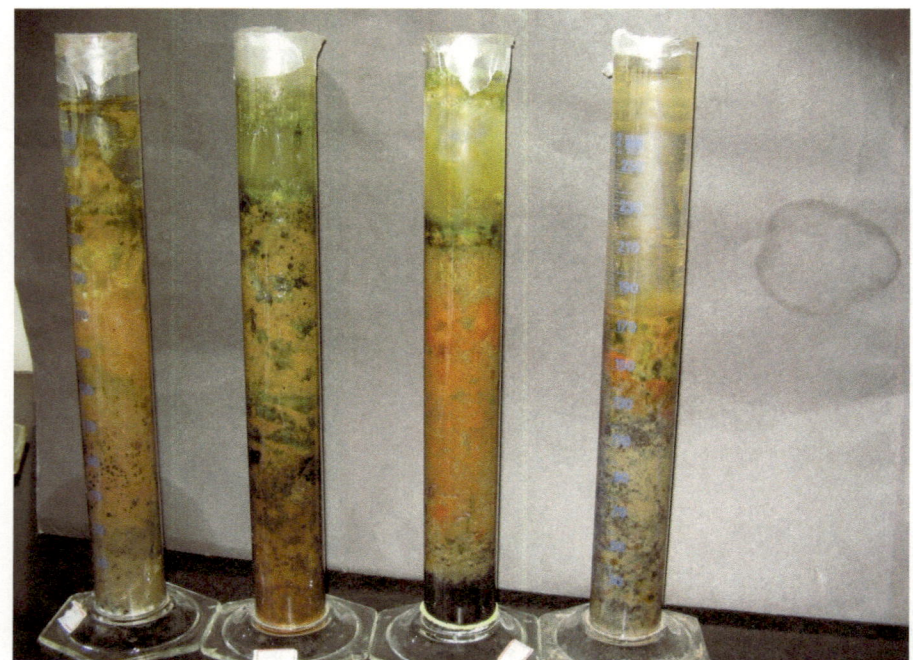

figure 9

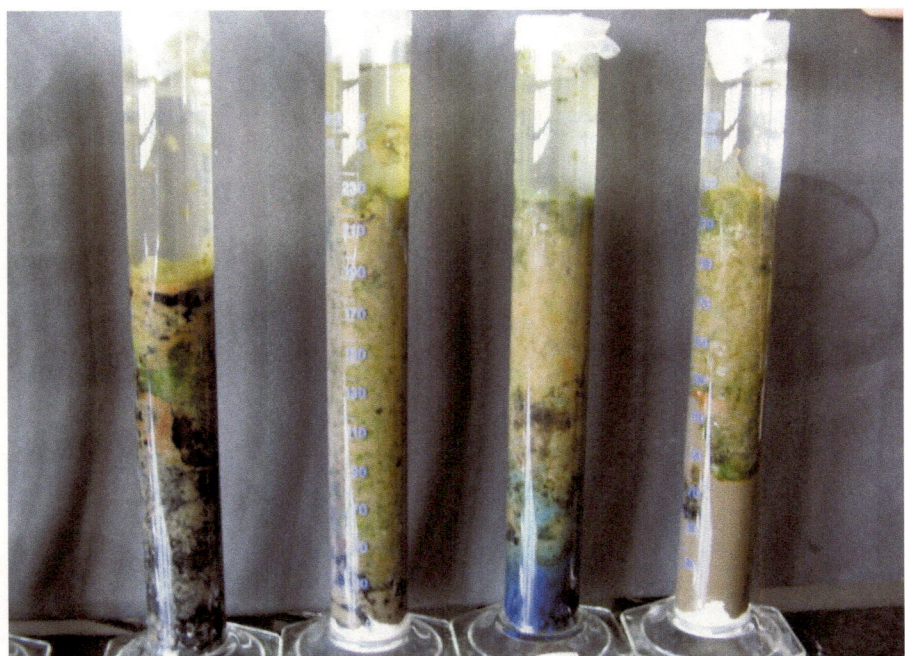

figure 10

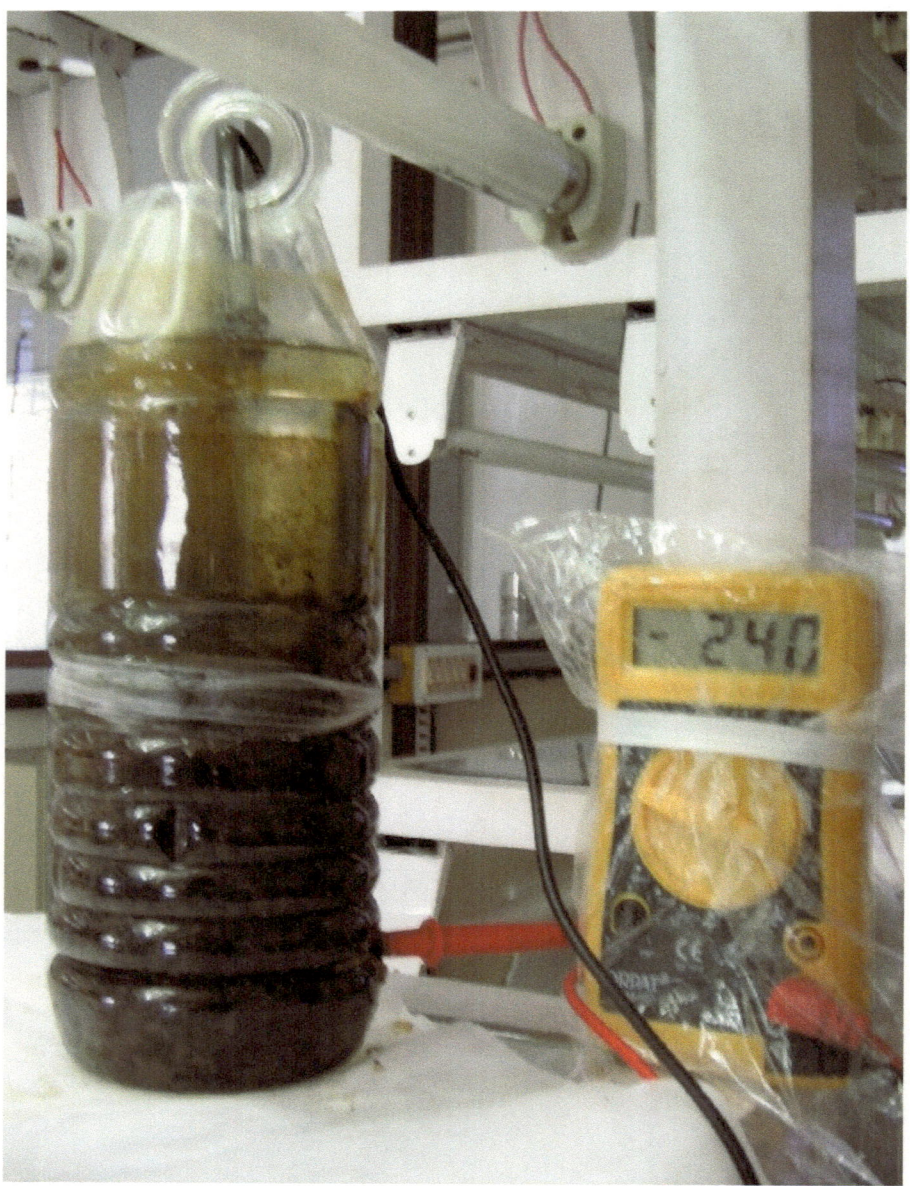

figure 11

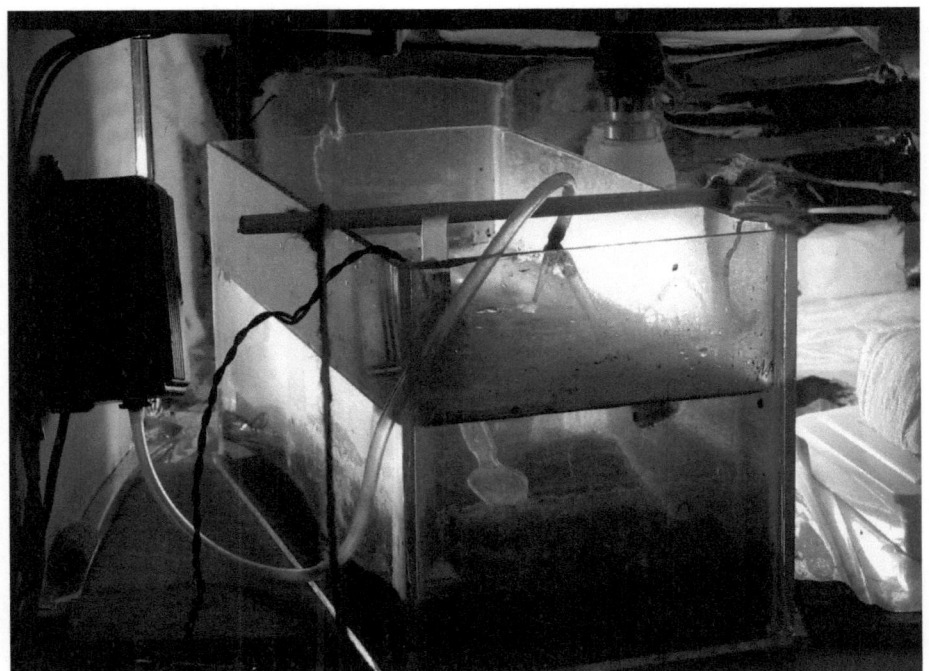

figure 12

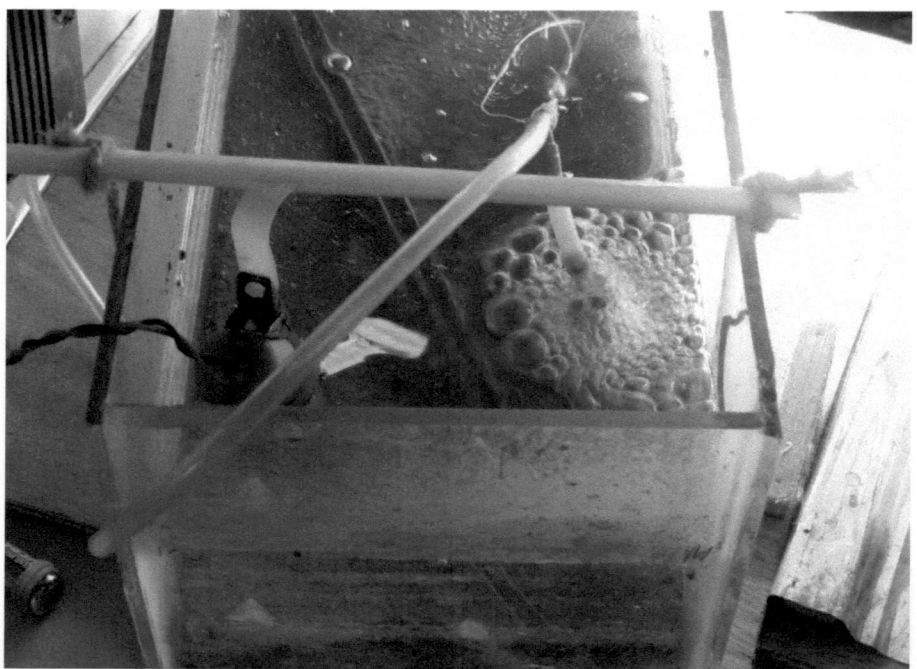

figure 13

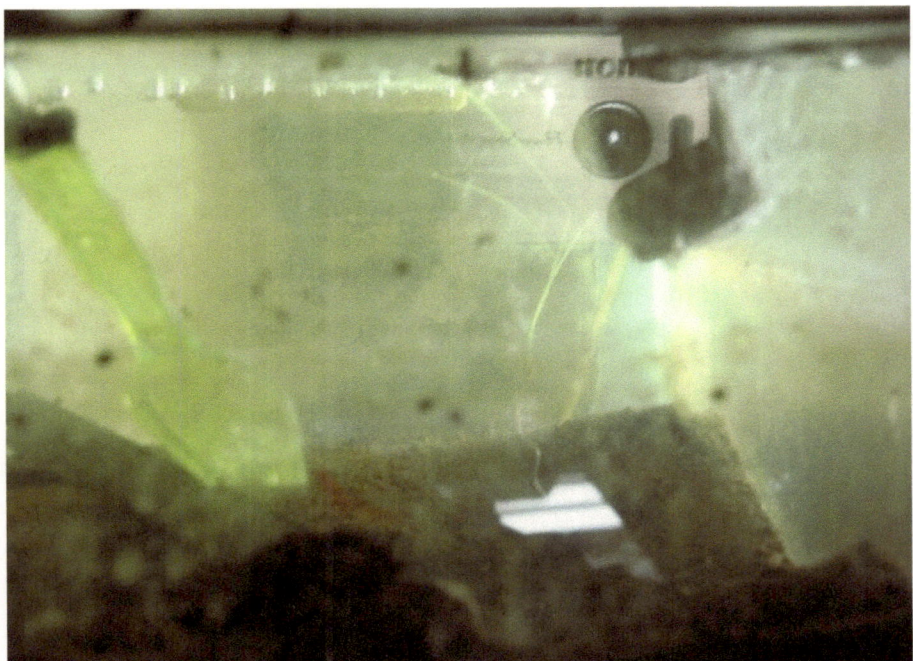

figure 14

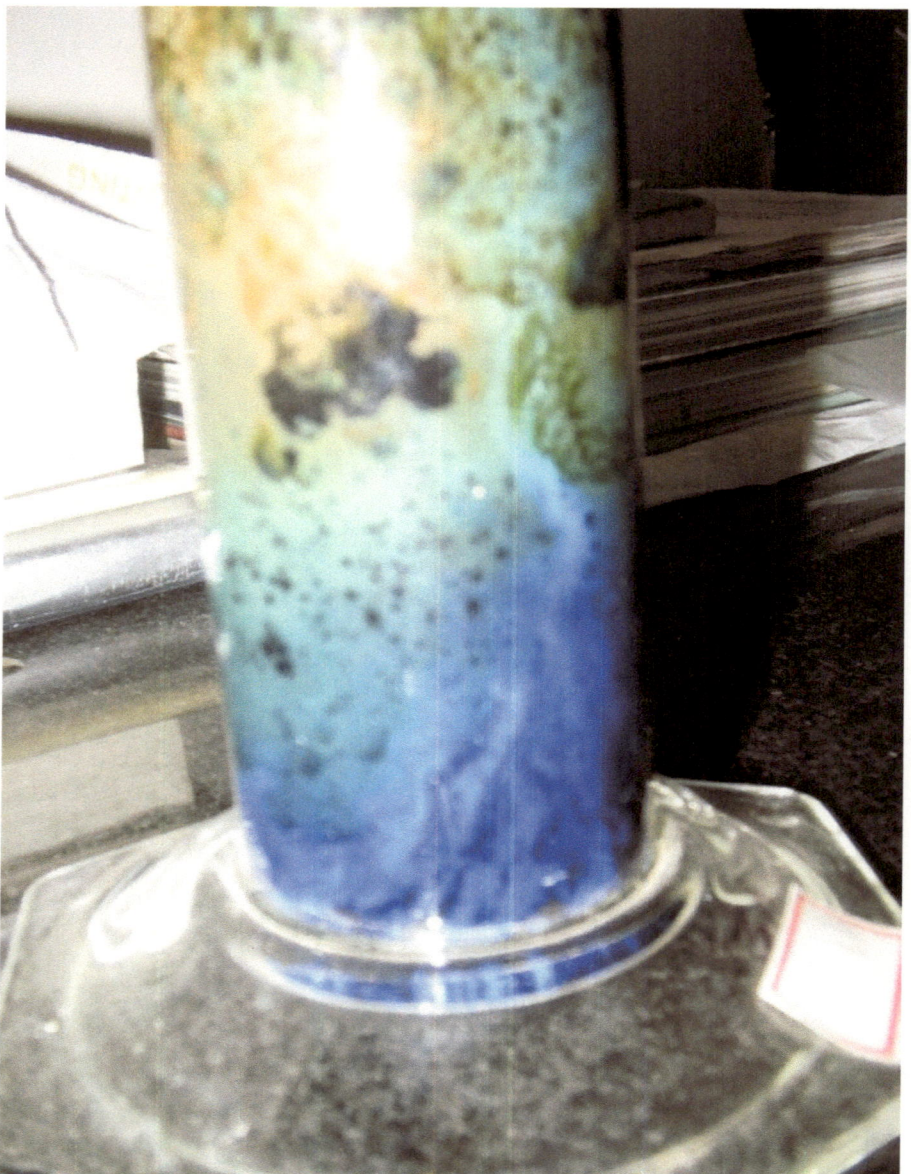

figure 15

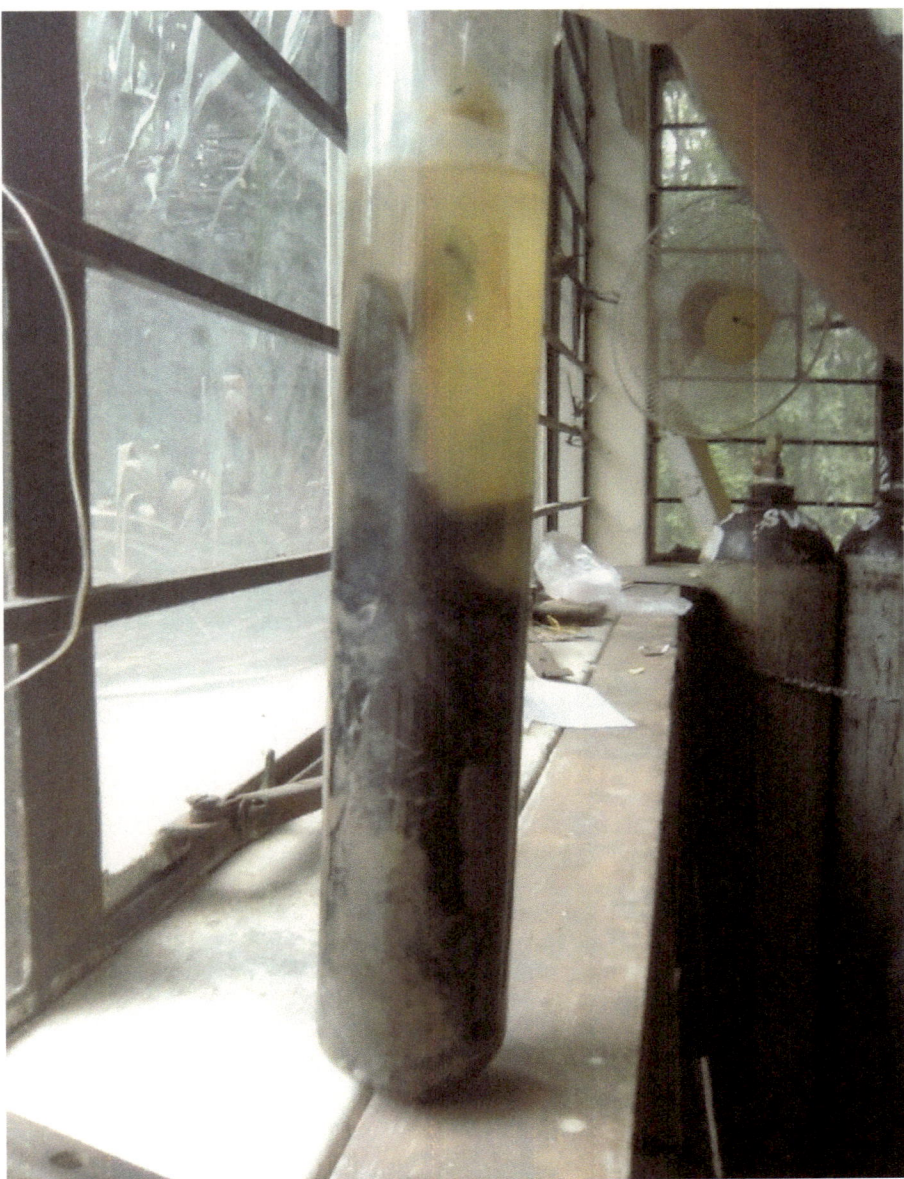

figure 16

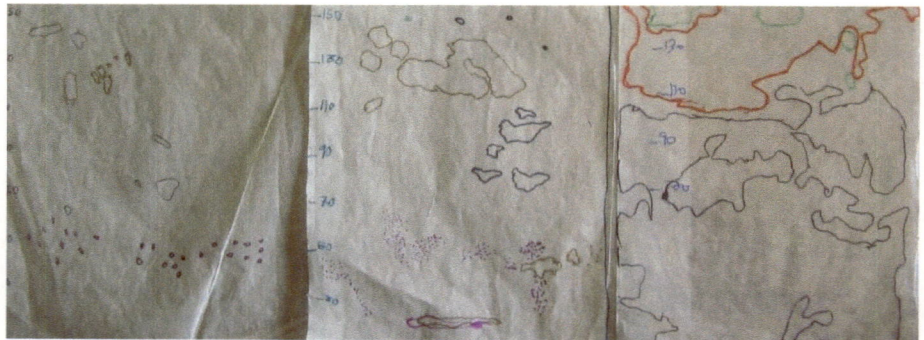
figure 17a

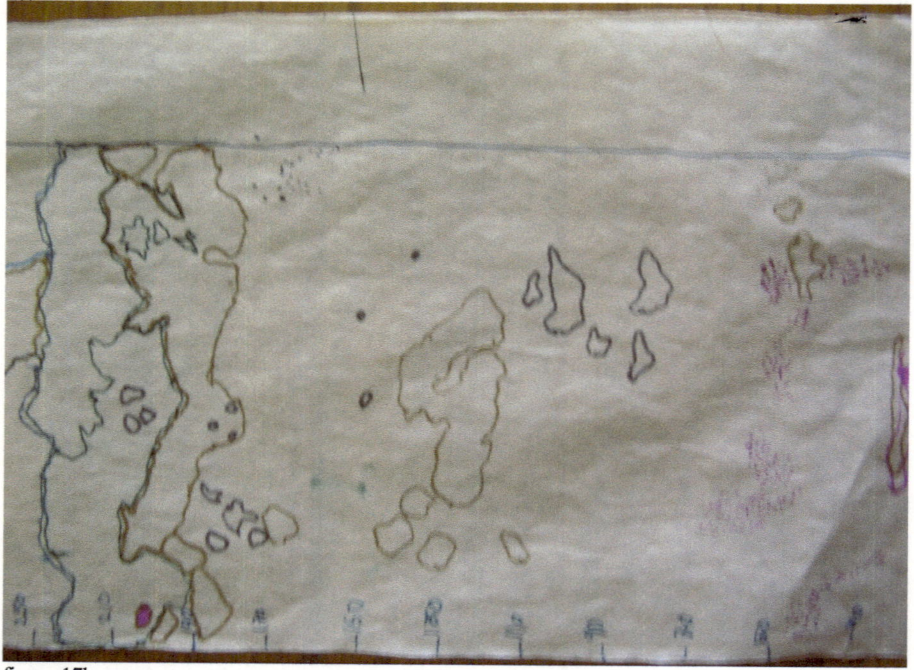

figure 17b

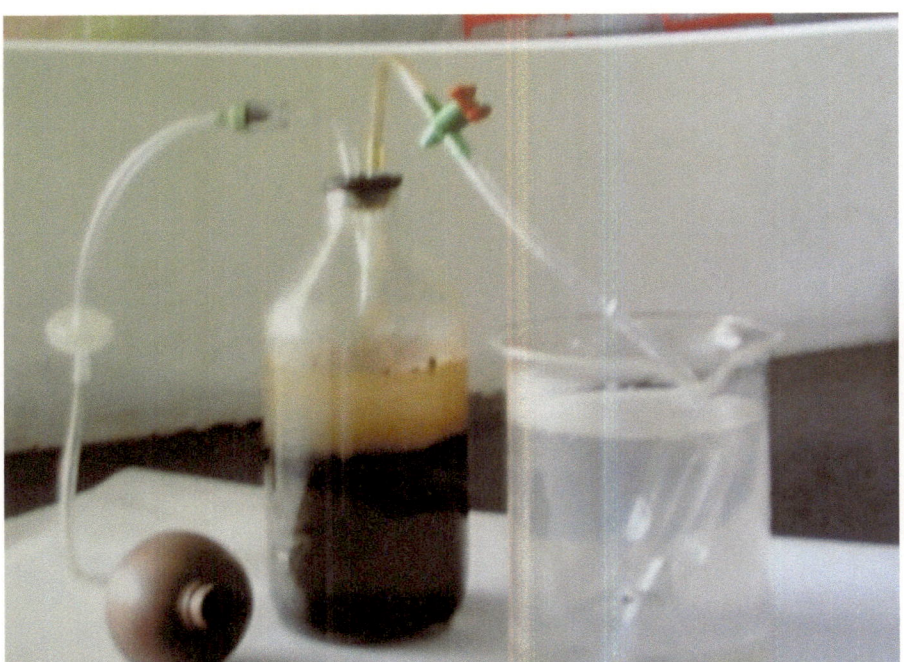

figure 18

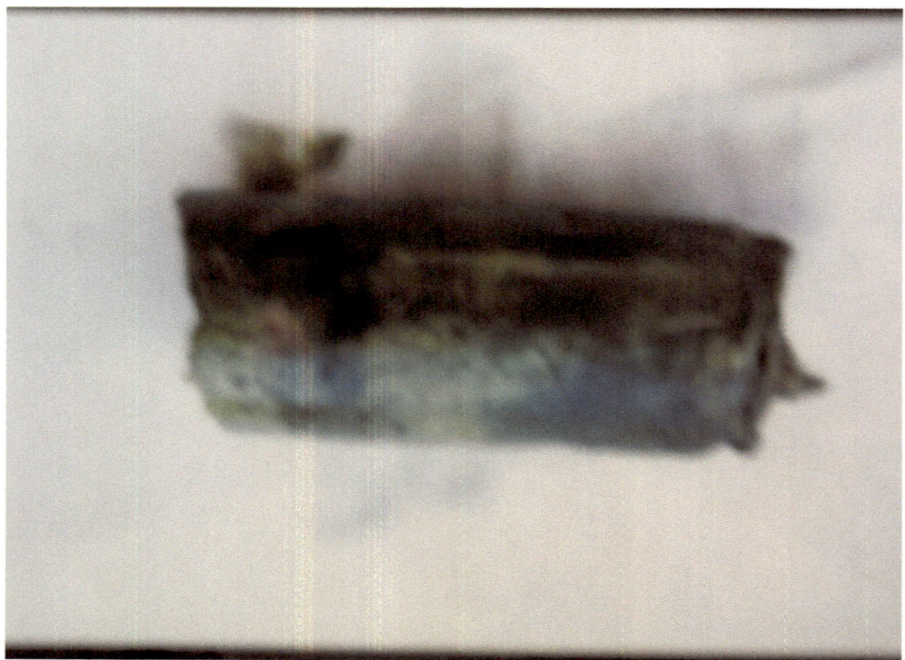

figure 19

Calculation

Similarly the the table showing biofilm pattern weight and time can be extended to any number of time and the weight predicted accordingly. Thus biofilm patterns can be predicted using regression equations and a perfect curve of biofilm weight versus time can be got (Table 1 and Table 2).

Table 1

Column number	Black Days 30, 60, 90*			Purple Days 30, 60, 90			Rust Days 30, 60, 90			Green Days 30, 60, 90			
1	0.035	***	0.529	0.058	0.074		0.207	0.577	0.189	0.135	0.788	0.	
2			0.275				0.239		0.369	0.490			
3			0.344				0.191	0.828	0.729	0.324	0.866	0.	
4			0.087						0.801			0.	
5	0.775	0.512	0.943		0.536	0.877	0.183	0.995	0.512	0.364	0.354	0.	
6		1.306	0.241		0.090	0.981			0.359				
7	0.824		1.566	0.015		0.263	0.061	0.805	0.548		0.888		
8		0.929		0.166								0.	
9		1.296	1.023					1.529	0.341		0.095	0.	
10	0.628	0.667	0.988	0.930	0.257		0.071	0.219	0.749	0.474	1.420		
11		0.808	0.794					0.281			1.045	0.	
12	0.331	0.609	0.773		0.054	0.550	0.341	0.081	0.016	0.021	1.145	0.	
13	0.300	0.759	0.477	0.072	0.030	0.090	0.300	0.110	0.238	0.192	0.696	0.	
14		0.047	0.388	0.029	0.089	0.265	0.274	0.350	0.204	0.250	0.857	0.	
5	0.340	0.721	0.890	0.020	0.129	0.043	0.336	0.095	0.675	0.079	1.201		
16	0.293	0.585	0.180		0.175	0.168	0.334	0.195	0.062	0.152	1.020	0.	
17	0.417	0.924	0.796				0.549	0.603	0.360	0.095	1.392	1.	
18	0.479	0.919	0.614				0.556	1.083	2.050	0.354	1.246	0.	
19	0.400	1.292	1.550				0.479	0.510	0.384	0.063	1.371	0.	
20	0.767	1.662	1.109	1.111				0.450	0.133		0.067		
21	0.295	0.250	0.435		0.038	0.116	0.742	1.277	0.456	0.766	1.024	0.	
22		1.096		0.402							0.551		
23	0.397	0.947	0.883		0.055	0.050	1.073	0.226	1.135	0.666	1.540	0.	
24	0.942	1.252	1.084				0.679	0.108	0.570		0.349	0.	
25	0.056	0.250	0.586					0.124	0.719	1.198	1.605	0.	
26		0.261	0.566	0.405			1.382	1.016	0.797	0.696	0.682	0.	
27	0.049	0.042	0.366				0.967	0.341	0.168	1.096	1.604	0.	
28	0.792	1.283	1.402				0.699	0.219		0.712	0.908		
29	0.831	0.957					0.513	0.554		1.010	1.103		

30	0.488	0.329					1.008	1.412		1.276	1.376	
31	4.553	0.656				0.211	1.398	0.534		1.035	0.942	
32 **	1.097						0.176			0.830		

* The data set can be generated for n number of days thus increasing the accuracy of the regression calculations. Herein the focus has been to generate a method to quatitate and to test it, so the data collection is left for further work. The same with the pattern prediction method, which gives the spatial distribution or biomass equivalents, a method has been standardised by which regression can be done to any given quantity of data set

**column 34 was for simulating pressure , column 35 was for simulating wind and waves (biofilm patterns were not measured for these) and column 36 for isolating methylotrophs for which the biofilm patterns were not traced over period of time

***gaps in the data indicate the disappearance of the pattern due to microbial succession

Table 2

Pattern prediction method					
Column 1 periodic readings	Rust colour pattern: (a grams)	e days	a^2	e^2	ae
1	0.206	30	0.423	900	6.195
2	0.577	60	0.333	3600	34.62
3	0.189	90	0.036	8100	17.00
Σ	0.972	180	0.411	12600	57.82

Pattern prediction Method

Mean $\bar{a} = \Sigma a / n = 0.342$

n = number of readings = 3

mean $\bar{e} = \Sigma e / n = 180 / 3 = 60$

$\sigma a = \sqrt{\Sigma a^2 / n - (\Sigma a)^2 / n} = \sqrt{0.411} / 3 - 0.324^2 = 0.179$

$\sigma e = \sqrt{\Sigma e^2 / n - (\Sigma e)^2 / n} = \sqrt{12600} / 3-60^2 = 24.49$

$r = \{ n \Sigma ae - (\Sigma a)(\Sigma e) \} / \{ \sqrt{n\Sigma a^2 - (\Sigma a)^2} \times \sqrt{n\Sigma e^2 - (\Sigma e)^2} \}$

$= \{3 \times 57.82 - 0.972 \times 180 \} / \{ \sqrt{3} \times .0411 - 0.972^2 \times \sqrt{3} \times 12600 - 180^2 \}$

$r = - 0.039$ (negative sign indicates that on drawing a graph both lines shall coincide in a downward nature)

a estimate $-\bar{a} = r \times \{\sigma a / \sigma e\} (e- \bar{e})$

a estimate $- 0.0324 = - 0.039 \times \{0.1792 / 24.49 \}(e- 60)$

substitute e = 90

a estimate = 0.333 g

e estimate $- \bar{e} = r \times \{\sigma e / \sigma a\} (a-\bar{a})$

e estimate $- 60 = -0.0039 \times \{24.49 / 0.1792\} (a - 0.3241)$

substitute a = 90

e estimate = g

Discussion

Most microorganisms are not yet cultured and classified because the specific microenvironments needed by them has never been achieved artificially in laboratory media. A specialised enrichment culture technique was discovered called as Winogradsky column, which is a tool capable of harbouring all microbes as they are. All the microbes are only maintained and according to the microenvironments that appear in the column, specific microbes grow successfully as visible biofilms. So the Winogradsky columns is limited to the few possible microenvironment conditions it is capable of simulating, and hence a few specific microbes that grow as visible biofilms. Though it simulates a pond microcosm, it is subjected to the lab environment, limiting its potentials only to demonstrating microbial succession and isolation and identification of some general microcosms.

The Winogradsky column was made use in this project to manipulate it in such a way as to create a unique set of environments as a preliminary step towards simulation of different environments. And it was shown that each manipulated microenvironment gave rise to a unique visible biofilm pattern. This culminated in the idea that if designing a Winogradsky that simulates any environment to the last detail, it could be of value to study microbes in biofilms. A Winogradsky column is a tool that simulates phenomena of microbial succession nutrient cycling, isolates few biofilm patterns and shows an intimate relationship between a localised environment and the resultant biofilm pattern.

The very fact that each biofilm pattern is unique to a specific location of water body by adjusting it and research can be conducted in a far away lab. To increase the simulation efficiency it was necessary to decide if altering the factors of a column alters the resultant biofilm patterns. It was found to be true by observing the biofilm patterns of many columns having variations in the factors. And to decide which factor causes which change, each column contained only one variation of a factor. Thus many columns were made.

One can get a regression curve from calculating quantitatively the biofilm patterns over a period of time using which one can tentatively predict the microenvironment and the biofilm pattern of the water body. And also with limited data available the gaps can be filled to create the whole curve of the growth pattern. The resulting biofilm patterns had to be kept in track for the purpose of analysing the relationship of environment. So Winogradsky maps were traced cut out and weighed. Thus the patterns were converted into mathematical data. This mathematical data was used to make predictions by using regression formulas. A regression formula can completely finish a curve got from scattered data. Thus, it minimised the tedious work of mapping and weighing frequently.

By simulating an environment "as it is", there is more chance to enrich all the microbes that find that environment suitable. Hence giving the uncultured microbes the best chances for its growth and hence identifying and classifying them.

The results also explain the reason why two ponds found in a same garden may never look the same in its biofilm pattern. And instead of making a normal Winogradsky column that never actually simulate the existing biofilm patterns one can make use of this modified column to simulate to a high degree. Thus the simulating potential of a normal Winogradsky column is very crude and generalised. Since each column of the many columns constructed by varying factors simulated the sample pond environment in some way because one among the variants of each factor matched the sample pond it is very tedious to make use of all the columns to simulate all factors with specific variations in a single column which can be really useful and easy to handle.

It is a simple observable fact that there are minute factorial changes that ultimately decide the biofilm pattern. A good simulator should be capable of making these minute factorial changes to bring about the exact conditions. It was necessary to manipulate each factor one at a time in one column at a time. This avoided confusions while interpreting the result that changing a factor or varying a factor brings about biofilm pattern changes. And it gave sufficient evidence to design the grand column. The reason for choosing only the pattern of biofilm and not the identification step was that a normal Winogradsky shows enough evidence of the intimate relationship to its localised microenvironment. Even in the columns constructed with factorial changes, one among them must partially simulate the actual sample pond. And its our hypothesis that the grand Winogradsky can simulate to the maximum.

Accidentally a form of evolution called high frequency gene transfer based evolution that takes place only in biofilms was observed. This evolution helped the columns having hard substrates to degrade them eventually in the form of dotted biofilm populations.

Time factor controls all the other factors. So the regression equations can help to decide the fate and condition for a water body, the survival conditions of the microcosms the resultant changes n the environment and the ageing phenomena of biofilms shown by sagging. Mapping the biofilm pattern changes in the columns was important for using the time factor and correlate and regress.

All these are sufficient evidence that the designed column can be a perfect simulator that grows microbes as they are in their environment. This serves as an answer to the long searched tool needed for exploration of microbial ecology with potent applications in biofilm technology. The hypothesis of making a grand simulation Winogradsky column can accurately simulate predict analyse and enrich any specific environment and the resultant biofilm pattern. There is hope to bring the simulation in silico also.

Winogradsky column can be used to isolate purpose based microbes. It can be used to study microbial biofilm interactions, analyse and predict biofilm patterns sums up in a new field theoretical microbiology. It can be used to harvest electricity. It can be used to simulate different microbe environments.

Acknowledgement

I kindly acknowledge the appreciation and support of Professor Lemke, University of Illinois, Springfield, Dr. N. Vijayaraj, National Institute of Health, Bethesda, Dr. Sengupta and Dr. Siddhartha of Indian Institute of Science, Dr. Sabitha Doraisamy and Arun, Dr.G.R. Damodaran College of Science, Dr V. Ramsundar Government Botanical Garden, Ooty, Dr. Hemant Chikarmane Marine Biology Lab, Woods Hole Oceanographic Institution, Massachusetts.

References

1. Anderson, Delia C, and Hairston, Hosalina V, The Winogradsky column and biofilms, models for teaching nutrient cycling and succession in an ecosystem, The American Biology Teacher, Vol. 61, No. 6, June 1999, pp. 453-459

2. Rogan, B., M. J. Lemke and M. Levandowsky. 2005. Exploring the sulfur nutrient cycle using the Winogradsky column. American Biology Teacher. 67:279-287

3. H.K. Pigage, The Winogradsky Column: A Miniature Pond Bottom, How-to-do-it, 239-240, The American Biology Teacher, Volume 47, No 4, April 1985

4. Madigan, M. T., Martinko, J. M. & Parker, J. (2000). Brock Biology of Microorganisms, 9th Edition. Upper Saddle River, NJ: Prentice-Hall.

5. Norbert Pfennig, Reflections of a Microbiologist, or How to learn from the microbes, Annual Reviews of Microbes, 1993, 47:1-29

6. Sylvia, D. M., Fuhrman, J. J., Hartel, P. G. & Zuberer, D. A. (1998). Principles and Applications of Soil Microbiology. Upper Saddle River, NJ: Prentice Hall.

YOUR KNOWLEDGE HAS VALUE

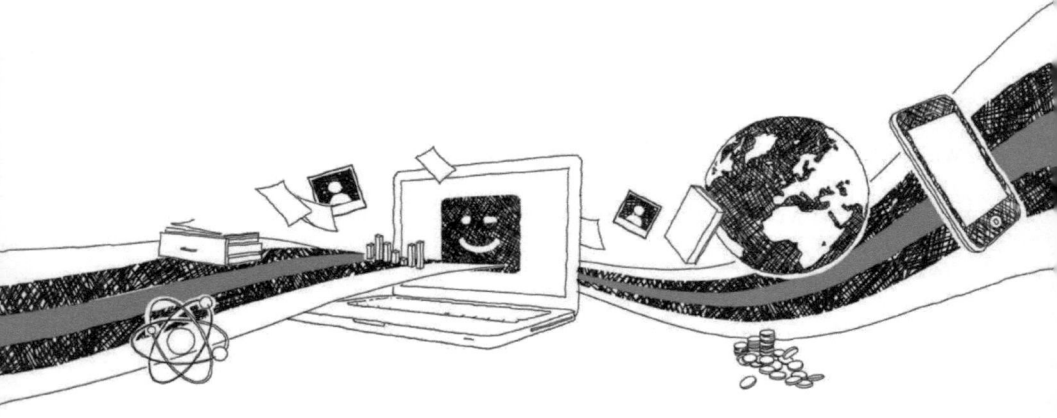

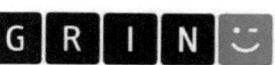